URBAN SKINNY NYC

Calorie Counted Meals at New York City's Hottest Restaurants

DANIELLE SCHUPP, RD

with Stephanie Krikorian

LYONS PRESS

Guilford, Connecticut
An imprint of Globe Pequot Press

To buy books in quantity for corporate use
or incentives, call **(800) 962-0973**
or e-mail **premiums@GlobePequot.com**.

Lyons Press is an imprint of Globe Pequot Press.

Text design: Sheryl Kober
Project editor: Kristen Mellitt
Layout artist: Mary Ballachino
Original maps provided by Compass Maps Ltd. © Morris Book
Publishing, LLC

Library of Congress Cataloging-in-Publication Data is available on file.

ISBN 978-0-7627-5080-1

Printed in the United States of America

10 9 8 7 6 5 4 3 2 1

Contents

Introduction

Eating out shouldn't stress you out. Ordering in a restaurant shouldn't be a calorie battle. There's a solu-
tion: *Urban Skinny NYC. Urban Skinny NYC* is the little
book you'll want to tuck into your Marc Jacobs bag
and take with you whenever you go out to eat. It's a
tiny portable calorie counter that helps you pick your
restaurants and choose your meals, so you can stay
on track with your Urban Skinny weight-loss program.

I'm Danielle Schupp, Reebok Sports Club/NY's
dietician. I've teamed up with writer and one-time cli-
ent Stephanie Krikorian to take a culinary trip through
Manhattan, all in an effort to keep you looking hot.
In this book we've given you restaurant choices for
power lunches, big dates, girls' nights out, and breakfast and brunch.

Stephanie and I went to every neighborhood,
spanning the culinary delights we all love to eat here
in the big city, putting together menus that will keep
your calories in check. We hit the restaurants that my
clients eat at over and over and polled some other
hip New Yorkers to find out where they'd like to eat
and still lose weight. We used Stephanie's dieter chal-
lenges ("There's no way I'm getting out of a Mexican
restaurant without having some guacamole!" or "I
can't eat red meat without one glass of Bordeaux"),
combined with my proven getting-lean strategies, to
help create some easy picks for you to order. We've
come up with 500- to 600-calorie meals for each restaurant entry, so you can go out and stay within your
calorie budget. For the majority of girls out there, a
500- to 600-calorie dinner is the target. But if you're
very active, on the tall side, or a guy, you can afford
a 700- to 800-calorie meal and still be in your losing
zone. So we've included a list of 100-calorie add-ons
at the back of the book to keep your budget in line.
The same applies if you're aiming for around 400
calories—shave 100 calories off your entree with portion control, or skip the extras.

Now, we couldn't possibly include every restaurant on the island of Manhattan, and we didn't get out to the boroughs, but we tried to give you a taste of something in every neighborhood, so you can make a choice and not be derailed by a night out. We also know that menus at a lot of restaurants change seasonally, so use your judgment when ordering.

Grab a copy of *Urban Skinny* for the entire weight-loss plan or log on to UrbanSkinny.com for extra tips and our blog. In the meantime, remember: Never deprive yourself of the things you like or you'll never successfully lose and keep off the weight. That's the backbone of *Urban Skinny*. We've given you lots of places to choose from including a "cupcake corner" and some awesome pasta picks! So grab your *Urban Skinny NYC* and hit the town, already! Live large, eat small!

Daily Caloric Chart

Note: If you are more than 100 pounds overweight, consult your doctor before starting any program.

*Minimum daily calorie intake for women is 1200.

		Sedentary	Moderately Active	Active	Very Active
WOMEN					
Height 5'0"–5'1"	Age 20–40 | above 160 lbs. add 100 calories	1200–1300	1400–1500	1600–1700	1800–1900
	Age 40–60 |	*1200	1300–1400	1500–1600	1700–1800
Height 5'2"–5'3"	Age 20–40 | above 170 lbs. add 100 calories	1300–1400	1500–1600	1700–1800	1900–2000
	Age 40–60 |	1200–1300	1400–1500	1600–1700	1800–1900
Height 5'4"–5'5"	Age 20–40 | above 180 lbs. add 100 calories	1300–1400	1500–1600	1700–1800	1900–2000
	Age 40–60 |	1200–1300	1400–1500	1600–1700	1800–1900
Height 5'6"–5'7"	Age 20–40 | above 190 lbs. add 100 calories	1400–1500	1600–1700	1800–1900	2000–2100
	Age 40–60 |	1400–1500	1500–1600	1700–1800	1900–2000
Height 5'8"–5'9"	Age 20–40 | above 200 lbs. add 100 calories	1500–1600	1700–1800	1900–2000	2100–2200
	Age 40–60 |	1400–1500	1600–1700	1800–1900	2000–2100
Height 5'10"–5'11"	Age 20–40 | above 215 lbs. add 100 calories	1600–1700	1800–1900	2000–2100	2200–2300
	Age 40–60 |	1500–1600	1700–1800	1900–2000	2100–2200

Sedentary: no specific exercise program, < 1 mile walking throughout the day, office job

Moderately Active: exercise program 3 times per week, office job; or no specific exercise routine but walks 2–3 miles per day every day

Active: exercises regularly 5–6 times per week, office job; or no specific exercise routine, walks 4+ miles per day @ 15 minutes per mile, 5–6 times per week

Very Active: exercises 6 days per week @ high intensity for 60+ minutes; or exercises more than once per day, e.g., triathletes, endurance athletes

Daily Caloric Chart

Note: If you are 100 pounds overweight, consult your doctor before starting any program. *Minimum daily calorie intake for men is 1500.

MEN		Sedentary	Moderately Active	Active	Very Active
Height 5'4"–5'5"	Age 20–40 | above 185 lbs. add 100 calories	1500–1600	1800–1900	2000–2100	2200–2300
	Age 40–60 |	*1500–1600	1700–1800	1900–2000	2100–2200
Height 5'6"–5'7"	Age 20–40 | above 195 lbs. add 100 calories	1600–1700	1900–2000	2100–2200	2300–2400
	Age 40–60 |	1500–1600	1800–1900	2000–2100	2200–2300
Height 5'8"–5'9"	Age 20–40 | above 210 lbs. add 100 calories	1700–1800	2000–2100	2200–2300	2400–2500
	Age 40–60 |	1600–1700	1900–2000	2100–2200	2300–2400
Height 5'10"–5'11"	Age 20–40 | above 220 lbs. add 100 calories	1800–1900	2100–2200	2300–2400	2500–2600
	Age 40–60 |	1700–1800	2000–2100	2200–2300	2400–2500
Height 6'0"–6'1"	Age 20–40 | above 235 lbs. add 100 calories	1900–2000	2200–2300	2400–2500	2600–2700
	Age 40–60 |	1800–1900	2100–2200	2300–1400	2500–2600
Height 6'2"–6'3"	Age 20–40 | above 250 lbs. add 100 calories	2000–2100	2300–2400	2500–2600	2700–2800
	Age 40–60 |	1900–2000	2200–2300	2400–2500	2600–2700

Sedentary: no specific exercise program, < 1 mile walking throughout the day, office job

Moderately Active: exercise program 3 times per week, office job; or no specific exercise routine but walks 2–3 miles per day every day

Active: exercises regularly 5–6 times per week, office job; or no specific exercise routine, walks 4+ miles per day @ 15 minutes per mile, 5–6 times per week

Very Active: exercises 6 days per week @ high intensity for 60+ minutes; or exercises more than once per day, e.g., triathletes, endurance athletes

Urban Skinny Starters: Tips for Eating Out

- Always order your salad dressing on the side.

- If you are having a glass of wine with your dinner, skip the bread, pasta, rice, or any other starch.

- Three ounces of chicken or steak is about the size of a deck of cards, and your fist is a cup of rice or pasta. Keep in mind, most restaurants serve 6 ounces of protein in an entree and a plate of pasta is usually more than 2 cups.

- You don't have to have two courses; one will sometimes do.

- A salad and an appetizer could make a good dinner portion, or split an entree with a friend.

- When in doubt, order grilled fish or chicken.

- Load up on veggies and salad.

- Keep the bread basket on the other side of the table.

- Drink lots of water.

- Be the first at your table to place your order so you don't cave to peer pressure.

- Try to decide ahead of time by looking at online menus and figuring out what you're going to order, so you're not tempted by something on the menu that's out of your calorie budget.

- Order things you like! Don't deprive yourself—just keep your portions in check.

Cocktail Hour Calories

Wine
6 ounces
150 calories

Champagne in Flute
100 calories

Vodka or Gin and Soda
1.5 ounces/shot
100 calories

Scotch, Whiskey
1.5 ounces/shot
100 calories

**Margarita on the
Rocks, Cosmopolitan,
Martini**
200–250 calories

Beer
150 calories per bottle

Light Beer
100 calories per bottle

**Port, Sherry,
Dessert Wine**
2 ounces
100 calories

**Mudslide or Piña
Colada**
800–1,000 calories

Frozen Margarita
16 ounces
500 calories

Latte
Small cup, 100 calories

Cappuccino
Small cup, 50 calories

Quick Tips for Ordering by Cuisine

Italian: Stick with red sauces, not oil or cream based. Opt for half-orders of pasta.

Greek: Lots of fish to choose from, but watch the pita and dips.

Japanese: Sushi isn't unlimited. The average piece is 50 calories.

Chinese: Most dishes can be ordered steamed, with sauce on the side.

Indian: Stick with the Tandoori and go easy on the naan.

Steak House: Think petite—a small piece of steak with veggies is okay, or go for fish.

Mexican: Pile on the salsa, not the guacamole.

Thai: Avoid anything with coconut and skip the Pad Thai.

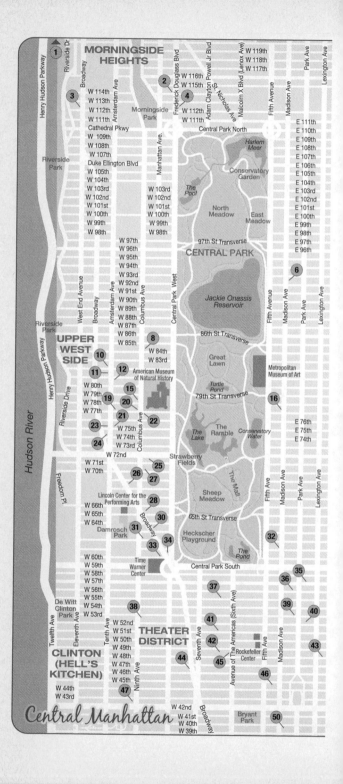

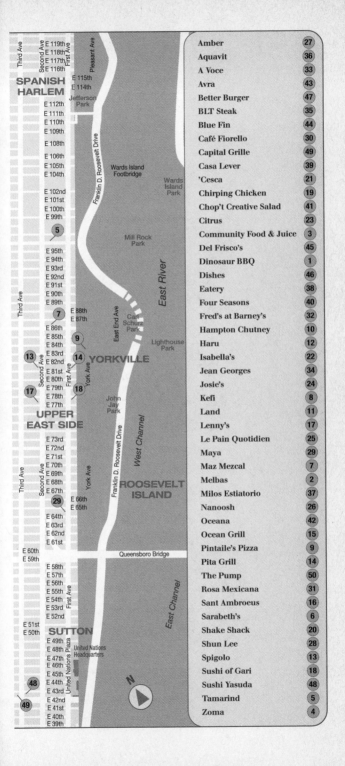

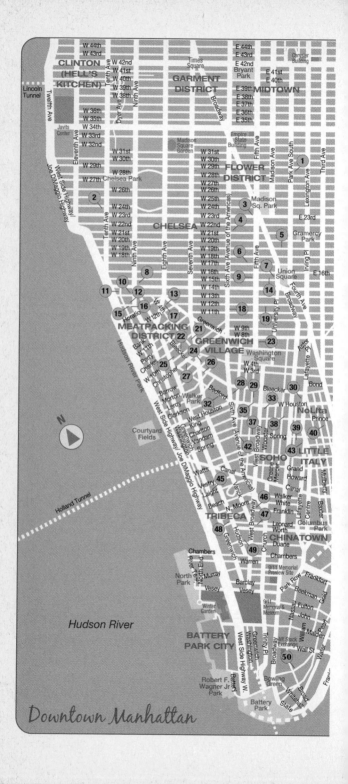

Downtown Manhattan

East River

United Nations Headquarters

Queens Midtown Tunnel

St Gabriel's Park

E 34th
E 33rd
E 32nd
E 31st
E 30th
E 29th
E 28th
E 27th
GRAMERCY
E 25th
E 24th

E 23rd

E 22nd
E 21st
E 20th
E 19th
E 18th
E 17th
Stuyvesant Square

STUYVESANT TOWN

E 20th

John J Murphy Park

E 14th
E 13th
E 12th
E 11th
E 10th
E 9th
E 8th
E 7th
E 6th
E 5th
E 4th
E 3rd
E 2nd
E 1st

ALPHABET CITY

Tompkins Square Park

John V. Lindsay/East River Park

EAST VILLAGE

East Houston
Hamilton Fish Park
Stanton
Rivington

LOWER EAST SIDE

Delancey
Broome
Grand
Hester
Canal

Corlears Hook Park

Seward Park
East Broadway

Franklin D. Roosevelt Drive

Manhattan Bridge

Empire-Fulton Ferry State Park

DUMBO

Cadman Plaza Park

BROOKLYN HEIGHTS

Montague

East River

Brooklyn Queens Expressway

Second Ave
First Ave
Franklin D. Roosevelt Drive
Ave A
Ave B
Ave C
Ave D
Essex
Ludlow
Clinton
Columbia
Baruch
Lewis

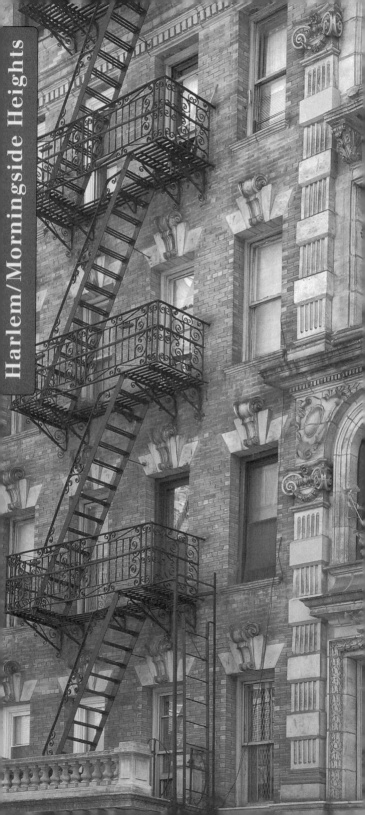

Community Food & Juice

Urban Skinny Bonus
There are lots of good brunch picks and seasonal organic options.

Urban Skinny Pick
The rice bowl is calorically priced just right. The veggies are raw, there's some sauce, and you can pick your protein. All in, it's around 400 calories, unless you choose salmon, and then it's more like 450 calories.

2893 Broadway between 112th St. and 113th St.
(212) 665-2800
www.communityrestaurant.com

Urban Myth: Skipping meals saves calories.

Urban Skinny: You may think skipping a meal helps, but when you finally sit down to eat dinner, you'll probably be starving and hit the bread basket hard so you'll not only make up the difference but eat more.

Dinosaur Bar-B-Que

Urban Skinny Heads-Up

We're not suggesting you tempt yourself by going here, but if your friends or date want to go, you can do it. There are options.

Urban Skinny Picks

Start with a chopped salad (it's only veggies) as a starter and leave the dressing off to save calories for something else.

AND

Shrimp Boil Platter for one, which has a ¼ pound of shrimp and comes with your choice of two sides. The shrimp will hit you for 140 calories, and pick some simmered beans for 50 calories, and baked beans for 150 calories.

That puts you at 350 calories, leaving room for *one* rib (200 calories) off someone else's plate.

OR

Try the Churrasco Chicken Sandwich, which is boneless, skinless, and grilled. Leave the mayo and cheese *off* the sandwich because there is already barbecue sauce in the mix. That's 450 calories. Add on a side salad and just count for dressing.

700 W. 125st St.
(212) 694-1777
www.dinosaurbarbque.com

Melbas

Urban Skinny Heads-Up

In general, soul food is not your best option for weight loss. There are so many temptations that are way over most people's calorie budget. But Melba's offers some healthy picks, keeping with the comfort food genre.

Urban Skinny Picks

Grilled Chicken (6–7 ounces precooked) is 200–250 calories.

OR

Grilled Salmon (6–7 ounces precooked) is 300–400 calories.

Add a vegetable salad and the jerk grilled shrimp appetizer for 125 calories; add 100 calories for dressing.

Urban Skinny Once-In-a-Whiles

A side order (about 1 cup) of Mac and Cheese is 400 calories. Have some greens and 100 calories' worth of salad dressing, but don't make this a habit.

300 W. 114th St.
@Frederick Douglass Blvd.
(212) 864-7777
www.melbasrestaurant.com

Zoma

Urban Skinny Bonus

Ethiopian food is a fun experience. You're not eating with forks, and you're likely trying things you may not have eaten before. It's great for sharing and quite filling.

Urban Skinny Note

All the food is served on a big spongy pancake for the entire table. Pick at lots of things, but watch the creamy sauces.

Urban Skinny Picks

Start with an appetizer of Lentil Salad served on endive for 50 calories each (4 in an order).

OR

Go for a simple Mixed Salad—just add calories for dressing.

Leanest combos:
Tibbs Wett is lean sirloin simmered in berbere spicy sauce. It's no more than 3 ounces of beef and has 300 calories for the serving.

Doro Wett is 2 small chicken drumsticks in berbere sauce at 125 calories each, 250 total.

Make sure to get some veggie picks in there as well—there are lots of vegetarian options.

Urban Skinny Tip

Injera bread is 150 calories for each little wrap. It acts as your utensil. Limit yourself to 1 injera bread and then eat with a fork (they'll bring you one if you ask for it).

Share with a girlfriend or a group and it's only about 600 calories for a satisfying and fun experience.

2084 Frederick Douglass Blvd.
@ 113th St.
(212) 662-0620
www.zomanyc.com

Urban Insight: When you cross the street, you look both ways. When you wake up in the morning, you brush your teeth. New life habit: When you order a salad, you get the dressing on the side. But hey, don't just pick it up and dump the whole thing on your salad—you ordered it on the side for a reason! Dip your fork in the dressing, then stab the lettuce.

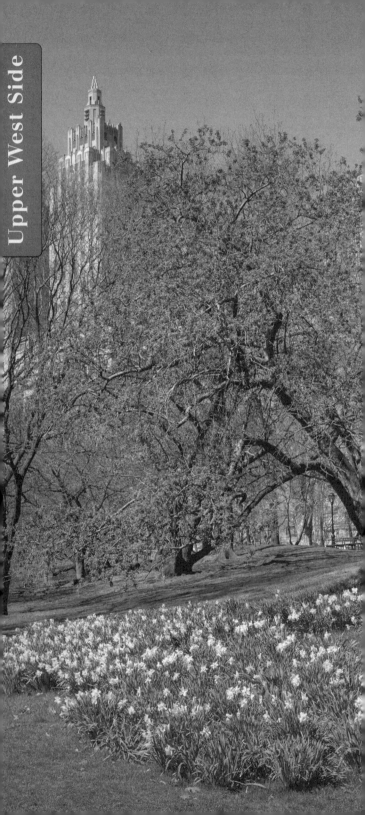

A Voce

Urban Skinny Bonus
There are many delish veggie sides to choose from so a starter doesn't have to be starchy or fried, it could be green!

Urban Skinny Picks
The pasta is good here, but the fish is a great option if you want a glass of wine. Branzino or poached halibut with an arugula salad to start (no dressing since there is ricotta in this salad) makes a nice 550 calorie choice.

Urban Skinny Pitfall
Bread and breadsticks. Need we say more?

10 Columbus Circle
(212) 823-2523
(Also @ 41 Madison Ave.; 212-545-8555)
www.avocerestaurant.com

Amber

Urban Skinny Bonus
Offers rolls with brown rice

Urban Skinny Picks
Amber Style Ceviche, 100–150 calories

Mango Vermicelli with 2 tablespoons of dressing, 200 calories

Chicken Satay, *no* extra peanut sauce, 150 calories

(A combo of a couple of these makes a great lunch or light dinner.)

Sushi Generation, 2 pieces of tuna and 1 salmon and yellowtail roll, 400 calories

Sushi and Sashimi for One is big enough for two, 750 calories.
    If you split this, order a side salad and a half an order of edamame and you'll be in the 550 calorie range.

1 Special Roll served with a side salad (#160–172 on menu), less than 500 calories

221 Columbus Ave., @ the corner of 70th
(212) 799-8100
(Also @ 1406 Third Ave., @ 80th St.; 212-249-5020)
www.ambercolumbus.com

Café Fiorello

Urban Skinny Picks

Go straight for the pizza—the crust is as thin as paper. The Signature Margherita Pizza, if you share and eat just half, will be under 400 calories.

AND

Add a green salad with dressing on the side for a 500-calorie meal.

Urban Skinny Pitfall

They put a very tempting bread basket on the table. Save your calories for the pizza.

1900 Broadway, between 63rd and 64th Sts.
(212) 595-5330
www.cafefiorello.com

'Cesca

Urban Skinny Bonus

You can ask for steamed veggies on the side and they'll honor this request.

Urban Skinny Appetizer Picks

Start with a few marinated Olives and 3 pieces Crudo, 120 calories.

OR

Mixed Green Salad, with 2 tablespoons of Parmesan Vinaigrette, 100 calories

Urban Skinny Entree Picks

Market Fish ala Livornese, 300 calories

Sea Scallops, 350 calories

Simply Grilled Tuna, 300 calories

Urban Skinny Heads-Up

If you really like foccacia, you can have one piece for l00 calories, but then be sure to skip the wine or any other starch. If you want wine, they pour a 6-ounce glass for l50 calories, so pick one or the other.

164 W. 75th St. @ Amsterdam
(212) 787-6300
www.cescanyc.com

Chirping Chicken

Urban Skinny Picks

Order a ½ chicken all-white-meat dinner and have it for 2 dinners, one breast each night. Without skin and wing, 250 calories per serving

AND

Side salad with dressing on the side, 100 calories

AND

Skip the pita and opt for *half* a baked or sweet potato

Total: 450–500 calories

Urban Skinny Add-On

Use the salsa for your potato or have 1 pat of butter, 75 calories.

355 Amsterdam Ave., between 76th and 77th Sts.
(212) 787-6631
www.chirpingchickennyc.com

Citrus

Urban Skinny Bonus
Lots of fish and sushi choices here, and they are all yummy.

Urban Skinny Picks
Make a meal of the Citrus Chopped Salad, but remember to get the dressing on the side and choose between the cheese and the avocado.

OR

Choose the shrimp or tuna entree, but eat only a half cup of the rice or potato side.

OR

Citrus Roll, two extra pieces of sashimi, and a green salad with the dressing on the side.

Urban Skinny Heads-Up
There are some great sides that accompany the fish, but they are often three servings in size, not one.

320 Amsterdam Ave.
(212) 595-0500
www.josienyc.com/citrus/citrus.html

Hampton Chutney

Urban Skinny Bonus
Gluten-free, great vegetarian options, sandwiches loaded with veggies

Urban Skinny Picks
Avocado, Fresh Tomato, Arugula, and Cheese with Chicken, 600 calories with dollop of non-peanut chutney

Urban Skinny Tip
Eat half (save the other half for tomorrow), and grab a piece of fruit for under 400 calories.

464 Amsterdam Ave.
between 82nd and 83rd Sts.
(212) 362-5050
www.hamptonchutney.com

Urban Myth: Losing weight fast is good.

Urban Skinny: The faster you lose it, the faster you gain it back. While it's true fast-paced New Yorkers want everything now, weight loss is the one thing in the Big Apple that does not happen in a New York minute.

Haru

Urban Skinny Bonus

You can ask for brown rice in Rolls and sushi, which is a daily fiber boost.

Urban Skinny Picks

Pick any two nonfried Rolls (8–12 small pieces)
Add on a Field Green Salad with 2 tablespoons of dressing (on the side)

OR

One Roll (any, nonfried type) and 4 pieces of Sushi, with a Field Green Salad (2 tablespoons of dressing on the side)

OR

Appetizer-size Edamame, Beef Negimaki, and a Field Green Salad (2 tablespoons of dressing on the side)

OR

Appetizer-size Black Cod Miso, Shrimp and Mushroom Shumai, Miso Soup, and Field Green Salad (2 tablespoons of dressing on the side)

Urban Skinny Extra

There are Rolls on the menu without rice, which helps save calories.

Urban Skinny Tip

If you are hungry, start with the Miso Soup to help fill you up, for less than 50 calories.

433 Amsterdam, between W. 80th and W. 81st
(212) 579-5655
(Also in Midtown @ 205 W. 43rd; 212-398-9810)
www.harusushi.com

Isabella's (Brunch)

Urban Skinny Heads-Up

This is a hot brunch spot and a challenge with all of the extra, yummy things that come with your meal, like a berry-mixed butter to eat with the bread—step away from that, but enjoy the complimentary drink. Make yours bubbly for 75 calories or a Mimosa for 125 calories.

Urban Skinny Picks

You can have the Eggs Benedict, just get the hollandaise on the side or ask for fat-free hollandaise. One tablespoon of the good stuff is 75 calories. Add that on top of the eggs, which already ring in at 350 calories.

OR

Egg White Omelette, 300 calories

OR

Seafood Cobb Salad, 300 calories without the dressing

Urban Skinny 100-Calorie Add-On

A side order of fruit

The Skinny

Remember brunch can be a little bigger meal (more than 500 calories) since you are combining breakfast and lunch.

359 Columbus Ave. @ 77th St.
(212) 724-2100
www.isabellas.com

Jean Georges

Urban Skinny Picks

Pick any two courses (an appetizer and an entree) with the exception of the tenderloin. These picks are each going to be about 200 calories. If you're really craving the tenderloin, have it for 450 calories, but just eat asparagus or another veggie side.

The Skinny

This is a hot restaurant for dinner, but we're giving you a fantastic choice for a sophisticated lunch, which in this case is a two-course choice that may not meet your financial budget but is great for your calorie budget.

1 Central Park West
(212) 299-3900
www.jean-georges.com

Urban Insight: Watch it—some places put butter on their beef or offer you sauces like béarnaise or au poivre, which can add anywhere from 100 to 400 calories to your cut of beef. Remember, you're not going to a steak house for the sauce. Dijon mustard is a great alternative for dipping; there's nothing to it. Steak sauces won't add up too quickly either. They're both low-calorie options as long as you don't drown your meat.

Josie's

Urban Skinny Bonus
Organic, soy cheese available, lots of seafood

Urban Skinny Picks
Seared Yellow Fin Tuna Burger served with mesclun greens, 450 calories

OR

Fresh Ground Natural Turkey Cheeseburger served with mesclun greens, 600 calories

Add a side of steamed veggies for no calories.

Urban Skinny Add-On
Fries are air-baked, 200 calories per "fist full." Skip the bun for the fries!

300 Amsterdam Ave.
@74th St.
(212) 769-1212
www.josiesnyc.com

Kefi

Urban Skinny Bonus

This place has some of the best fish on the Upper West Side.

Urban Skinny Picks

Start with a Kefi salad with the dressing on the side for 150 calories. The swordfish, branzino, or seabass are all great choices at 300 calories each. They aren't served with a starch side so feel free to order the bulgur salad and share with a girlfriend.

OR

Share the meze platter with one pita and opt for the octopus appetizer: total intake 550 calories. Be sure to dip don't dunk into the tzatziki.

Urban Skinny Heads-Up

It's safest to avoid most of the appetizers here, which are calorie-laden.

505 Columbus Avenue
(212) 873-0200
www.KefiRestaurant.com

Land

Urban Skinny Bonus
Great for ordering in or takeout

Urban Skinny Picks
One or two Veggie Steamed Dumplings, 50 calories each

AND

Wok Basil Chicken or Shrimp. Scoop protein and veggies out of sauce. It is flavorful enough—there is no need for extra sauce. Six ounces of protein in each entree: chicken, 300 calories, or shrimp, 250 calories 1 cup of rice, 200 calories

450 Amsterdam Ave., between 81st and 82nd Sts.
(212) 501-8121
www.landthaikitchen.com

Urban Myth: You can eat all of your calories in one meal.

Urban Skinny: Spacing out your calories between small meals every three or four hours throughout the day helps rev up your metabolism.

Le Pain Quotidien (Breakfast)

Urban Skinny Bonus
Organic ingredients when possible, stone ground flour; calorie counts on site

Urban Skinny Picks
Organic Soft Boiled Egg with Bread, 290 calories
Organic Steel-cut Oatmeal, 200 calories and a good source of fiber

Urban Skinny Add-On
Small Fresh Fruit Bowl, 110 calories

Urban Skinny Pitfall
Avoid the 1,100-calorie Baker's Basket.

60 W. 65th St.
@ Columbus Ave.
(212) 721-4001
www.lepainquotidien.com

Urban Myth: Some foods are taboo.

Urban Skinny: Live a little. No foods are good or bad. The key is portion control and never overspending your calories. If you can't live without a donut, have one, but not three. Don't be greedy. A glazed Krispy Kreme donut is only about 200 calories.

Nanoosh

Urban Skinny Bonus
Organic, whole-wheat pitas, and you can add fresh veggies to any dish

Urban Skinny Picks
Green Salad with Citrus and Walnut Dressing: carrots, raisins, walnuts, and arugula with 2 tablespoons of dressing, 150 calories

AND

Hummus Chicken—eat about 2–3 ounces of chicken and ¼ cup of hummus and only one pita, 400 calories

Urban Skinny Pitfall
This dish is served with 2 pitas and 1½ cups of hummus, so save the extra for another meal or split with a friend.

2012 Broadway
@69th St.
(212) 362-7922
www.nanoosh.com

Ocean Grill

Urban Skinny Bonus
3 servings of veggies in the Urban Skinny Pick

Urban Skinny Picks
Ocean Chopped Salad with Feta and Olives, 1 table-spoon of dressing on the side, 200 calories

AND

Go for any of the 6 types of "simply grilled" 7-ounce (precooked) portions of fish. The white fish picks, 250 calories; or salmon, 350 calories. Pick a Bokchoy and Mushroom side dish for 50 calories and Lemon Emulsion or Soy-Ginger Vinaigrette side for 50–100 calories.

384 Columbus Ave.
@78th and Columbus
(212) 579-2300
www.oceangrill.com

Rosa Mexicana

Urban Skinny Bonus
Guacamole is rich in heart-healthy oils. There is also a gluten-free menu.

Urban Skinny Picks
Ensalada de la Casa (house salad) with dressing on the side, 100 calories

Ceviche de Huachinango (marinated red snapper and shrimp), 100 calories

Mariposa de Huachinango (roasted red snapper) brushed with chili sauce and salsa on the side, 350 calories

OR

Salmon en Manchamanteles (Salmon with tropical fruit mole) served over black beans with zucchini and roasted corn, 500 calories

Urban Skinny Add-On
Pomegranate Margarita, 200 calories—so you can only eat half the salmon entree if you're having one of these.

Urban Skinny Pitfall
The guacamole bowl is 600–800 calories before you even add in the chips.

61 Columbus Ave.
@62nd St.
(212) 977-7700
www.rosamexicano.com

Shake Shack

Urban Skinny Heads-Up

Entering this place requires strength and discipline. It's a minefield of good stuff packed with calories. But it can be done. Just decide in advance what you're having and don't deviate. The burgers are 4 ounces. The Single Hamburger is 370 calories. The Single Shack Burger is 470 calories.

Urban Skinny Pitfalls

The mushroom burger is not your best choice here— it's deep-fried and covered in cheese. And, not that a custard smoothie sounds like it could be a healthy choice, but avoid it—it's loaded with saturated fat and calories.

**366 Columbus Ave., between 77th and 78th Sts. (646) 747-8770
(Also in Flatiron @ Madison Square Park, E. 23rd and Madison Ave.; 212-889-6600)**

Shun Lee

Urban Skinny Bonus
Lots of veggies available

Urban Skinny Picks
Steamed Veggie Dumplings, 150 calories

Hot and Sour Cabbage, 50 calories

Szechuan Bouillabaisse, 150 calories

Half an order of Heavenly Fish Filet, 350 calories

Spicy Steamed Prawns with the sauce on the side, 200 calories

Add 100 calories for each ¼ cup of sauce.

**43 W. 65th St., between Columbus and CPW
(212) 595-8895
www.shunleewest.com**

Urban Insight: When walking in New York City, twenty city blocks is a mile, which translates to 100 burned calories. Four crosstown blocks is a mile. Start walking. If you don't have blocks to measure, grab a cheap pedometer or order one on your iPhone. If you clock 2,000 steps, that's approximately a mile. You might find the pedometer keeps you motivated as you see how your walking adds up throughout the day.

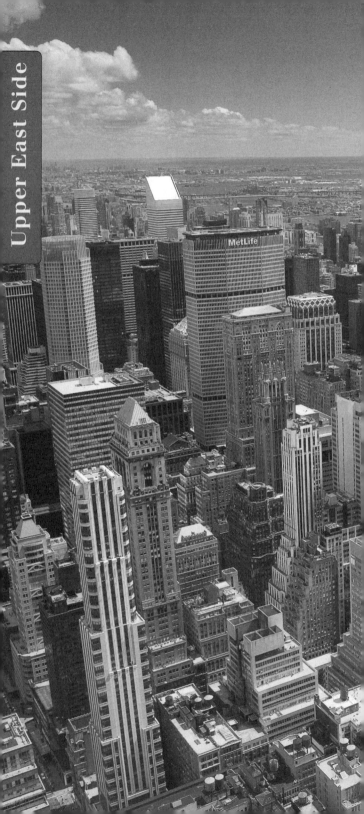

Lenny's

Urban Skinny Picks

Sandwich: Create your own roasted turkey or grilled chicken with avocado *or* mayo, whole grain bread, and pile on the veggies, 450–500 calories.

Salad: Make your own with mesclun or spinach and add as many veggies as you like since they are essentially calorie free.

Ingredients from Group B, 50 calories each

Ingredients from Group C, 100 calories each

Ingredients from Group E, chicken, shrimp, tuna, or turkey, 100 calories

Salmon, 150 calories

Stay clear of the mayo-based salads.

Be sure to add a protein to your salad in order to stay full.

1481 2nd Ave.
@ 77th St.
(212) 288-5288
www.lennysnyc.com

Maz Mezcal

Urban Skinny Bonus

The guacamole is a smaller portion than other New York Mexican restaurants. It's made from only 1 avocado. The total bowl is only 400 calories. *But* they serve 3 types of salsas to dip chips in, so there is no need to even order the guacamole.

Urban Skinny Starters

Ceviche de Camaron (shrimp with avocado salsa), 150 calories

Sopa de Pollo (chicken and veggies in a clear broth), 150 calories

Ensalada Verde (green salad with avocado), 2 tablespoons of dressing, 200 calories

Urban Skinny Entree Picks

Huachinango Capistrano (red snapper in a pico de gallo sauce with corn), 350 calories

Camarones en Salsa Verde (shrimp in a green sauce with veggies), 350 calories

Urban Skinny Heads-Up

Skip the rice and beans served with the entrees.

316 E. 86th St., between 1st and 2nd Aves.
(212) 472-1599
www.mazmezcal.com

Pintaile's Pizza

Urban Skinny Bonus
Paper-thin whole-wheat crust with wheat germ and fresh mozzarella

Urban Skinny Picks
Veggie-topped pies, 350–400 calories per slice

Chicken or Gobble, 425 calories per slice

1573 York Ave., between 83rd and 84th Sts.
(212) 396-3479
(Also @ 26 E. 91st St., between 5th and Madison
Aves.; 212-722-1967)
www.pintailespizza.com

Urban Myth: Carbs are evil.

Urban Skinny: Anybody who stays lean long-term eats things like sweet potatoes, bananas, pasta, and sandwiches. Try to eat whole grains, but it's all about portion control. A half of a whole-wheat bagel is about 250 calories.

Pita Grill

Urban Skinny Bonus
Offers great fresh salads with a selection of regular and low-fat dressings

Urban Skinny Picks
The Pita Grilled Salad with grilled chicken and eggplant over mesclun, with dried cranberries and feta cheese. Order the Light Roasted Red Pepper Vinaigrette on the side. Order the small salad, which has 4–5 ounces of chicken and 450 calories. Add 35 calories per tablespoon of dressing used.

OR

The turkey burger is a great size—4-ounce portion of meat—so with the bun it has 400 calories. Order with the garden salad with dressing on the side; add 50 calories per tablespoon of regular dressing, and 25–35 calories per tablespoon of light dressing.

1570 1st Ave., between 81st and 82nd Sts.
(212) 717-2005
www.orderpitagrill.com

Urban Insight: With salad dressing, don't confuse ounces for tablespoons. Ask at lunch counters how much is in each little dressing container. The standard size is 2 ounces, which, for the record, is 4 tablespoons. So a 2-ounce container of vinaigrette will cost you 200 calories; creamy dressing is 300 calories.

Sant Ambroeus

Urban Skinny Bonus
Nice seafood picks with an Italian twist

Urban Skinny Entree Picks
Try the chef's fresh fish of the day, with a side of greens and a glass of wine for under 500 calories.

Urban Skinny Light Pick
Insalata di Nettuno is a mixture of lump and king crab meat with sliced fennel and orange for 150 calories, and opt for 2 tablespoons of dressing on the side, for just 250 calories. Add a slice of bread for 100 calories. Perfect for lunch.

1000 Madison Ave., between 77th and 78th Sts.
(212) 570-2211
www.santambroeus.com

Sarabeth's (Brunch)

Urban Skinny Bonus
Cooks eggs with nonstick spray upon request

Urban Skinny Picks
Baby Bear Hot Porridge, with milk and honey on the side, 300 calories before honey, 60 calories per tablespoon with it

OR

Egg white omelets with veggies and a touch of cheese

Omelets are on the large side, so count 350–400 calories. Opt for the English muffin instead of the muffins, croissants, or scones for only 120 calories.

OR

Eggs Benedict, hollandaise on the side, 330 calories without the hollandaise, 75 calories for each tablespoon of hollandaise you dip

Urban Skinny Add-On
Mimosa or Bloody Mary, 150 calories

1295 Madison Ave. between 92nd and 93rd Sts.
(212) 410-7335
www.sarabethseast.com

Spigolo

Urban Skinny Bonus

Girls, if you want pasta, this is the place. It offers the perfect pasta portion! Olives are placed on the table instead of the taboo bread basket.

Urban Skinny Picks

The portion size is perfect at 2 ounces. The pasta is listed as a primi course, but enjoy it as your entree. There are typically 5 different pastas to choose from, all no more than 400 calories!

If you're not in the mood for pasta, get the Grilled Shrimp appetizer over farro as a main and pair it up with the delicious Shaved Celery Salad. Order dressing on the side, of course, for a total of 500 calories.

1561 2nd Ave.
@81st St.
(212) 744-1100
www.spigolonyc.com

Sushi of Gari

Urban Skinny Bonus

Sushi is a great way to stay on track because there's no bread basket to grapple with and you don't go to a sushi restaurant for the wine list. There are also no really yummy desserts to resist.

Urban Skinny Starters

Oshitashi (boiled spinach), 50 calories

Hijiki Salad (black seaweed and watercress), 100 calories

Edamame (boiled soybeans), 200 calories

Ebi or Kani Shumai (steamed crab or shrimp dumplings), 50 calories each

Miso Soup, 25–50 calories

Urban Skinny Entree Picks

Sushi regular or Tuna of Gari, 8 pieces sushi and 1 tuna roll, 600–650 calories

It may be better to either order pieces of sushi or sashimi (50 calories per piece of sushi and 25–35 calories per piece of sashimi) or share an order of regular sushi since it is a large portion.

402 E. 78th St., between 1st and York Ave.
(212) 517-5340
(Also @ 347 W. 46th St., between 8th and 9th Aves.; 212-957-0046)
www.sushiofgari.com

Tamarind

Urban Skinny Starters
House salad with ginger-lemon dressing on the side, with 2 tablespoons, only 100 calories

Urban Skinny Heads-Up
If you must have bread, stick with a piece of Roti for about 100 calories.

Urban Skinny Entree Picks
Chicken Tandoori

OR

Tikka Kebab

OR

Tandoori shrimp

150 calories per deck of cards measure (includes extra for the oil it might have cooked in)

Urban Skinny Pitfall
Indian food is sauce heavy—ask for yogurt if you need something to cool the spice, but watch for the other heavy ones.

1679 3rd Ave.
@ 94th St.
(212) 410-9400
(Also @ 424 Amsterdam Ave., between 80th and
81st Sts.; 212-712-1900)
www.rhgnyc.com

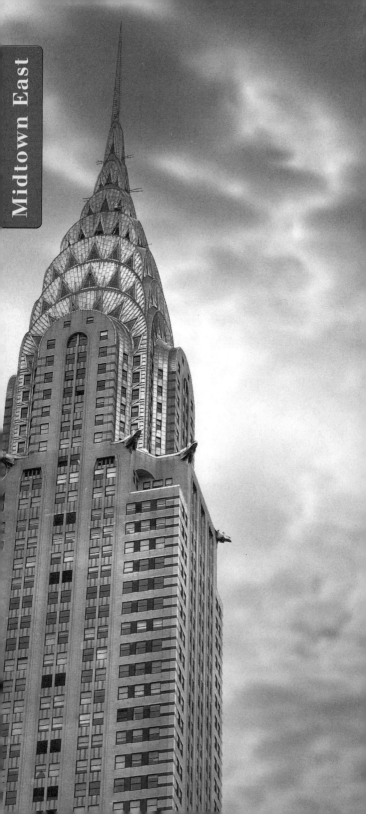

Aquavit

Urban Skinny Bonus

You can get a light lunch and a shot of heart-healthy omega-3 oils! This is a great place to take clients for a light business lunch.

Urban Skinny Picks

Opt for the bistro for a more casual dining experience and also where you can order a la carte. Start with the Gem Field Green Salad with 2 tablespoons of vinaigrette on the side instead of the caesar dressing, 100 calories.

Scandinavian Bouillabaisse, 250 calories

Slice of bread, 100 calories

65 E. 55th St.
@ Madison Ave.
(212) 307-7311
www.aquavit.org

Urban Skinny Bonus

This is one of the hottest new places in town. It's for the fabulous, and fortunately its fish options are plentiful.

Urban Skinny Pick

Start with the Spitiki Simple Salad, with the dressing on the side, and order a deboned 1-pound fish, which will amount to 6 ounces. Order some steamed greens and a glass of wine for under 500 calories.

141 E. 48th St.
(212) 759-8550
www.avrany.com

Urban Insight: The medical world has long known the health benefits of a traditional Mediterranean diet, which typically consists of whole grains, plenty of veggies, and heart-healthy olives and olive oils.

BLT Steak

Urban Skinny Heads-Up

Step away from the popovers—they are 350 calories each.

Urban Skinny Picks

The Chopped Salad with 2 tablespoons of dressing on it, 150 calories

Spiced Tuna or Branzino, for 250 calories. If you need a sauce, opt for the soy-citrus, which adds 50 calories.

OR

Half portion of the 12-ounce filet mignon, 250 calories

Poached String Beans, 50–100 calories

106 E. 57th St., between Park and Lexington Aves.
(212) 752-7470
www.bltsteak.com

Capital Grille

Urban Skinny Tip
This is a great lunch spot because they offer smaller portions than at dinner.

Urban Skinny Bonus
There are lots of entree salad options. Just dip, don't dunk, your dressing, which of course is ordered on the side.

Urban Skinny Entree Picks
Any of these with 4 tablespoons of dressing will equal less than 500 calories.

Seared Salmon Salad, 300 calories, if you skip the wonton croutons

OR

Salad with Chilled Shrimp, 200 calories

OR

Lobster Salad, 200 calories (request sour cream on the side; 1 tablespoon, 50 calories)

OR

Sesame Seared Tuna, 250 calories

Urban Skinny Heads-Up
You're only getting 4 tablespoons of dressing on your salad because it's an entree size. Otherwise, stick to under 2 tablespoons.

155 E. 42nd St. (Chrysler Center)
(212) 953-2000
(Also @ the Time-Life Building, 120 W. 51st St.;
212-246-0154)
www.capitalgrille.com

Casa Lever

Urban Skinny Bonus
A prix-fixe lunch means two nicely portioned courses.

Urban Skinny Appetizer Picks
Carciofi: artichoke, parmesan, and arugula

OR

Casa Lever Salad, 150 calories (skip the dressing since there is cheese)

Urban Skinny Entree Pick
Choose any of the white fish courses for 250–300 calories.

Urban Skinny Add-On
If you skip all the starch on the table, have a glass of wine for 150 calories.

390 Park Ave.
@ 53rd St.
(212) 888-2700
www.casalever.com

Dishes (Workday Breakfast or Lunch)

Urban Skinny Bonus
There are lots of organic foods, including a nitrate-free roasted turkey (nitrates may increase your risk for cancer), olive oil- and canola oil-based dressings, and 100 percent whole-wheat rolls. And they deliver!

Urban Skinny Breakfast Picks
Steel-cut Irish Oatmeal prepared with water (other oatmeals are prepared with whole milk). Top with fresh fruit and toasted walnuts.
Small, 300 calories
Large, 400 calories

OR

Organic Egg White Omelet, with veggies and 2 slices of whole-wheat toast, 400 calories

Urban Skinny Lunch Picks
Nitrate-free, roasted turkey with cheddar on 7-grain bread, request mayo on the side, 450 calories (mayo is 100 calories per tablespoon)

OR

They have a great make-your-own salad bar. So pile on the veggies, and add either Ancho Roasted Salmon or Blackened Chicken Breast. Count 150 calories per "tong" for chicken/salmon, cheese, avocado, nuts, and 50 calories per "tong" for beans or corn. Order dressing on the side and toss it yourself. A 2-ounce container of oil-based dressing is 200 calories.

6 E. 45th St.
@ 5th Ave.
(212) 687-5511
www.dishestogo.com

Four Seasons

Urban Skinny Bonus
Be seen in the scene at this hip power lunch spot.

Urban Skinny Business Lunch Pick
Go with the Ahi Burger with Spicy Ginger Mayo on the side and skip the fries, 400 calories.

99 E. 52nd St., between Park and Lexington Aves.
(212) 754-9494
www.fourseasonsrestaurant.com

Fred's at Barney's New York

Urban Skinny Bonus
Nice light fare perfect for ladies who lunch

Urban Skinny Picks
For a light lunch, try the Tuna Tartar served over mixed greens but request dressing on the side. Use 2 tablespoons of dressing and it's only 250 calories. Add a piece of bread for 100 calories for a perfect 350-calorie lunch.

The Madison Avenue Salad is a signature salad made up of mixed veggies, beans, and topped with imported tuna. Request dressing on the side and use 4 tablespoons, since it's a large salad, for 500 calories.

660 Madison Ave.
@61st St.
(212) 833-2200
www.barneys.com

Maya

Urban Skinny Starters
Ceviche de Atun, 150 calories

Urban Skinny Entree Picks
Three-Chile Crusted Tuna with Blood Orange Salsa,
400 calories

OR

Mole Poblano, 400 calories

Urban Skinny Heads-Up
If you must have one of their delicious margaritas on
the rocks (200 calories), make sure to adjust your
food intake or split a starter and entree with a friend.

1191 1st Ave.
between 64th and 65th Sts.
(212) 585-1818
www.richardsandoval.com/mayany

The Pump

Urban Skinny Bonus
Calories are now listed on the website, which helps you choose your meal ahead of time.

Urban Skinny Pick
The Rookie Steak Burger: Made with 93 percent lean fresh ground beef served on a whole-wheat pita. A great burger for only 450 calories and only 20 calories more than the turkey burger, pizza style, which is 430 calories.

Urban Skinny Heads-Up
When it comes to burgers, size does matter. Not all burgers are this well-sized.

275 Madison Ave.
@ 40th St.
(212) 697-7867
www.thepumpenergyfood.com

Sushi Yasuda

Urban Skinny Bonus
Japanese food is salty but low in calories!

Urban Skinny Picks
Miso Soup, 50 calories

AND

Sushitake, which is 8 pieces of sushi and a half roll, 550 calories

Urban Skinny Tip
Oshitashi (boiled spinach with shaved dried bonito) has essentially no calories and is a good source of vitamin K, folate, and vitamin A.

204 E. 43rd St., between 2nd and 3rd Aves.
(212) 972-1001
www.sushiyasuda.com

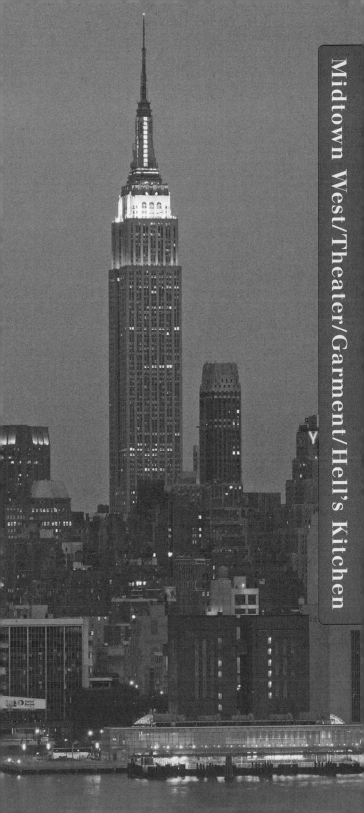

Better Burger

Urban Skinny Bonus

Burgers are offered in 2 portion sizes, ⅓ pound and ½ pound (precooked), and they're made from Brandt Natural beef, which comes from cows fed a vegetarian, corn-based diet for more than 365 days without hormones or the use of antibiotics. They're served on whole-wheat buns.

Urban Skinny Picks

Go for the ⅓-pound burger on a bun, 450 calories.

Add a garden salad of greens with 2 tablespoons dressing on the side, 100 calories.

If you want the fries, drop the bun for a total of 550 calories—the fries are air-baked at 270 calories per serving.

587 9th Ave., between 42nd and 43rd Sts.
(212) 629-6622
www.betterburgernyc.com

Blue Fin

Urban Skinny Bonus
Sushi picks make Blue Fin an easy choice.

Urban Skinny Picks
Blue Fin Tuna Burger with Ginger and Avocado is 350 calories, but request the spicy aioli on the side. Substitute a mixed green salad with dressing on the side for the fries.

OR

Seafood Cobb Salad, with shrimp, crab, avocado, and ruby red grapefruit, 300 calories

OR

Lobster Salad with Hearts of Palm and Avocado and Citrus Vinaigrette, 300 calories

Be sure to request all dressings on the side and add 50 calories per tablespoon that you use.

W Hotel, Times Square
1567 Broadway
@ 47th St.
(212) 918-1400
www.bluefinnyc.com

Chop't Creative Salad

Urban Skinny Bonus

You can mix multiple types of lettuce in your salad, and all salad dressings here are homemade and have heart-healthy olive or canola oil.

Urban Skinny Picks

Build a salad, keeping in mind that each ingredient is measured with ¼ cup measuring cup and some-times it's heaping, making things like the turkey or chicken more like ⅓ cup and therefore 75 calories. Add cheese for 100 calories and dried fruit or half a portion of nuts (2 tablespoons) for an additional 100 calories. As usual, request dressing on the side. The dressing container here is 3 ounces, unlike other salad restaurants, where it is typically 2 ounces. So if it's full of vinaigrette, *just* the dressing is 300 calories if you eat it all; low-fat is 150 and fat-free is 100 calories.

Salad is served with a wedge of tortilla, which will ding you for 50 calories.

145 W. 51st St., between 6th and 7th Aves.
(212) 974-8140
www.choptsalad.com

Del Frisco's

Urban Skinny Starters

House Salad with dressing on the side (2 tablespoons is 100 calories)

Urban Skinny Entree Picks

6-ounce Filet Mignon or Blackened Salmon is 350 calories if you skip the potato. Taste the Chocolate Mousse for about 150 calories or have a glass of wine.

Total: 500 calories

OR

Maine Lobster Salad with Citrus Vinaigrette (4 tablespoons dressing), 400 calories

Urban Skinny Pitfall

Steak houses can be tricky when you have the steak and the heavy sauced sides. It all adds up pretty quickly.

1221 Avenue of the Americas
@ 49th St.
(212) 575-5129
www.delfriscos.com

Eatery

Urban Skinny Bonus
Eatery is a great brunch pick with some reasonable calorie choices.

Urban Skinny Heads-Up
Avoid the air-puffed treats that land on your table when you sit down for dinner, and the brunch cakes that arrive for brunch.

Urban Skinny Picks
Scrambled Egg White Tortilla with Organic Cracked Wheat Salad, Sweet Corn, Queso Fresco, and Salsa Verde, 450 calories

OR

Japanese Egg White Omelet with Shiitake Mushroom, Tofu, Japanese Eggplant, Plum Glaze, and Pickled Cucumber Salad, plus a slice of dry wheat toast, 350 calories

OR

Irish Oatmeal with Fresh Berries, Currants, Toasted Pistachios, and Cinnamon Syrup, 400 calories
    Request syrup on the side and drizzle on only 1 tablespoon.

798 9th Ave., between 52nd and 53rd Sts.
(212) 765-7080
www.eaterynyc.com

Milos Estiatorio

Urban Skinny Bonus

This place serves up plenty of veggies and fruits with the three-course prix-fixe menu.

Urban Skinny Starter

Tomato Salad with Feta Cheese, 150 calories

Request dressing on the side. The salad is small and feta has plenty of flavor, so you really only need 1 tablespoon of vinaigrette.

Urban Skinny Entree Pick

Whole White Fish of the Day, simply grilled, but be sure to request that they go light on the oil, 250–300 calories.

You can order fresh fruit here for an additional 125 calories as your dessert, or have a glass of wine instead.

125 W. 55th St., between 6th and 7th Aves.
(212) 245-7400
www.milos.ca

Oceana

Urban Skinny Pick

Always choose the white fish, which comes in
6-ounce portions. The menu changes seasonally,
but you can always get the mixed Green Salad with
dressing on the side, 2 tablespoons, 100 calories,
and white fish. Striped bass is a standard.
Fish entrees, 300–400 calories

Urban Skinny Tip

Avoid the four-course prix fixe—go a la carte.

120 West 49th St.
McGraw-Hill Building
(212) 759-5941
www.oceanarestaurant.com

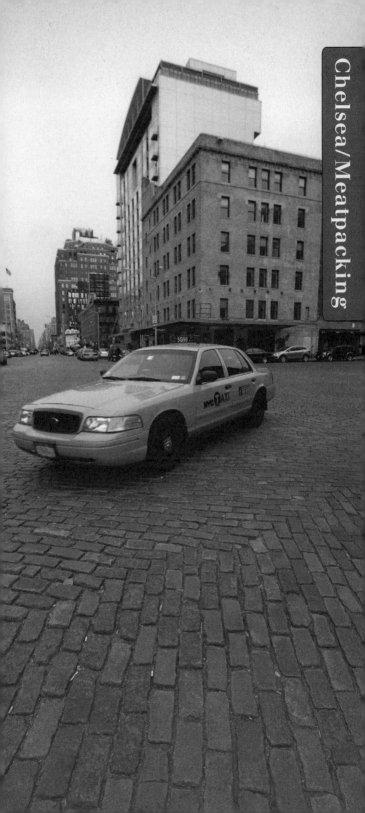

Chelsea/Meatpacking

BLT Fish

Urban Skinny Heads-Up

If you eat a Cheddar and Chive Biscuit, you've almost eaten your entire dinner, because it's 300–350 calories.

Urban Skinny Picks

The whole fish for one is 8 ounces. They typically have Dover sole, branzino, and lobster, so just the fish is going to be 300 calories based on the serving size here. Skip the optional sauces and you can add something like wine or a salad to your dinner for 500 calories.

The salmon is higher in calories—around 450–500 calories. Dishes are served with tiny sides of veggies, greens, or beans.

Urban Skinny Light Pick

Combine two appetizers to make one meal. Try the Arugula Salad with Pecorino and 2 tablespoons of vinaigrette for 250 calories, and maybe some Yellow Fin Tartar for an additional 150 calories. If you leave the dressing off your salad, you might have room for all or some of that biscuit and still come in at 500–600 calories.

21 W. 17th St., between 5th and 6th Aves.
(212) 691-8888
www.bltfish.com

Les Halles

Urban Skinny Picks
Two appetizers, one meal

Dive into the Classic French Onion Soup for 400 calories and have the Mixed House Salad with 100 calories in dressing.

OR

Go for the Les Halles Fitness option in a pick-and-choose menu.

Six-ounce precooked portion of your choice served with vegetables (can be steamed)

Steak, 300 calories

Chicken, 200 calories

Fish or Shrimp, 150 calories

Urban Skinny Tips
Dip your steak in Dijon instead of heavy sauces like béarnaise.

Add a glass of Chablis or Bordeaux and you're out the door for less than 500 calories.

Urban Skinny Pitfall
Sauces, escargot drenched in butter, and French bread and butter. Don't derail your day for a plate of frites.

411 Park Ave. S, between 28th and 29th Sts.
(212) 679-4111
www.leshalles.net

Mesa Grill

Urban Skinny Picks

Spicy Tuna and Salmon Tartar appetizer (3-ounce portion served with 1 ounce of chips), 250–300 calories

AND

Shrimp Tamale, 200 calories, with Sophie's Chopped Salad with dressing on the side,100 calories (before dressing)

OR

Stick with a fish entree (7 ounces precooked). The menu changes but always has several white fish choices, which are 300 calories, or 400 calories if there is a starch on the plate.

Urban Skinny Pitfalls

Salmon is a staple on the menu, but don't forget it can be as much as 450 calories for an order.

Avoid a la carte sides, since most are pretty rich and they cost extra.

102 5th Ave.
(212) 807-7400
www.mesagrill.com

Paradou

Urban Skinny Heads-Up

This menu, like many, changes seasonally. Charcuterie and cheese are always on the menu. An ounce of cheese is between 75–100 calories and so is an ounce of sausisson.

Urban Skinny Picks

Start with the Herb Salad with Oven-Roasted Tomato for about 150 calories, if you include some dressing. Go with fish, grilled, or split a grilled beef dish with a friend—fish will be under 250 calories, and beef will be around 350 calories for half of what they serve you.

Get a side of Haricot Verts for 100 calories and ask them to steam, instead of sauté.

Urban Skinny Pitfall

Stay clear of the duck dishes, pâtés, and the seasonal cassoulet.

8 Little W. 12th St., between 9th St. and Washington Ave.
(212) 463-8345
www.paradounyc.com

Pastis

Urban Skinny Picks

Opt for the Chicken Pallaird for any meal—it's available for lunch, brunch, or dinner—for a total of 350 calories. It's 6–8 ounces of protein. Be sure to order the mustard vinaigrette on the side.

OR

Split the Croque-Monsieur or Croque-Madame with a girlfriend and add a simple salad and call it a day, for 500–600 calories.

Urban Skinny Tip

If you must have the Onion Soup, make it your entree, because it's 400 calories. Pair it up with a simple salad with dressing on the side.

9 9th Ave., on the corner of Little W. 12th St.
(212) 929-4844
www.pastisny.com

The Red Cat

Urban Skinny Picks

Make two apps your meal. Try the Sautéed Calamari Stew or Mussel dish because it's a tomato-based stew and is about 300 calories. Add an order of the Quick Sauté of Zucchini for another 250 calories.

You then have plenty of room to try the Potato and Lobster Pierogies, 100 calories each.

Urban Skinny Pitfall

As tempting as they may be, try to avoid the Tempura Fried Green Beans with Honey Mustard Sauce. They're a house specialty, but a huge portion that will add up very quickly. And once you eat one, it's hard to stop.

227 10th Ave., between 23rd and 24th Sts.
(212) 242-1122
www.theredcat.com

Urban Myth: Always make your appetizer a salad.

Urban Skinny: Ceviche, shrimp cocktail, and lump crab are great options, too. If you want a salad before an entree, make it a vegetable salad only. If you get the beet and cheese or tomato and mozzarella or anything with nuts, you need to make that your entire meal—not your starter.

Scarpetta

Urban Skinny Heads-Up
The spaghetti here is to *die* for, but they cheese and butter it for you, so split it with someone else.

Urban Skinny Entree Picks
Half an order of the Spaghetti with Tomato and Basil is 300 calories to start. Follow with a piece of grilled fish for a 500-calorie dinner.

OR

Black Maccheroni Pasta with Seafood. Eat all the seafood and half the pasta for 500 calories.

355 W. 14th St., between 8th and 9th Aves.
(212) 691-0555
www.scarpettanyc.com

Spice Market

Urban Skinny Bonus
This is a great place for sharing with a lot of healthy choices.

Urban Skinny Starter
Start with the Market Salad as a filler before you even get going, because it will have no calories before dressing, and 100 calories if you use just 2 table-spoons—and it will fill you up.

Urban Skinny Options to Share
Chicken Skewers with 5 skewers per order, 5–6 ounces, 200 calories, but be sure to dip, don't dunk, in lime sauce.

Pick at some Steamed Mussels, with a typical 1-pound order being 400 calories.

The Shaved Tuna has about 100 calories per order.

Shrimp Dumplings in a Lemongrass Broth are 50 calories per dumpling.

Urban Skinny Heads-Up
Be mindful—you can have a bunch of different things, but keep track as you eat. Don't eat all the mussels, all the dumplings, a few skewers, and drinks, and think since you're sharing, the calories don't add up.

403 W. 13th St.
@ 9th Ave.
(212) 675-2322
www.spicemarketnewyork.com

STK

Urban Skinny High-Five
This place is on our hot list because their website says it has a waistline-conscious menu.

Urban Skinny Bonus
Bread is served only upon request, and they'll steam your veggies if you just ask.

Urban Skinny Picks
Garden Salad, 100 calories (dressing on the side)

OR

Jumbo Lump Crab with Melon, 150 calories

OR

Scallop Ceviche, 100 calories

OR

Make all three your meal and have a glass of wine for under 500 calories.

If you want steak, opt for the 6-ounce (precooked weight) strip or filet mignon for 350 calories, and one pick from the apps list above. And remember, a good steak doesn't need sauce. Don't waste the calories.

**26 Little W. 12th St., between 9th Ave. and
Washington St.
(646) 624-2444
www.stkhouse.com**

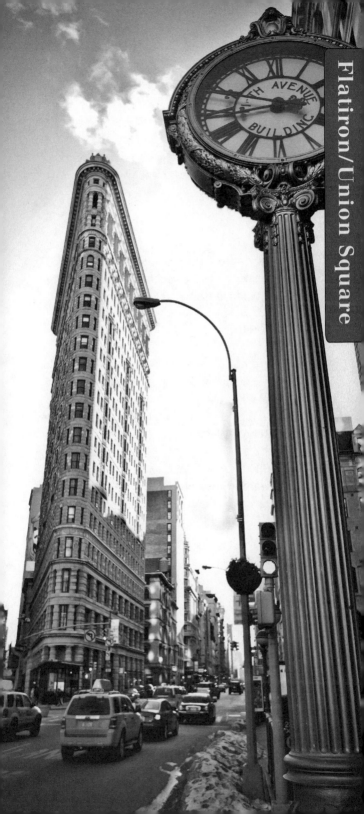

Blue Water Grill

Urban Skinny Bonus
They offer simply grilled fish.

Urban Skinny Picks
Blue Water Grilled, Chopped Salad (no dressing because the feta and olives provide plenty of flavor), 150 calories

AND

Typical fish entree, 6 ounces precooked, 200 calories
Simply grilled comes with a vegetable side, so opt for the spinach or tomatoes for 100 calories.

Total: Salad, fish, and veggie sides, 500 calories

Urban Skinny Heads-Up
That Cobb Salad that looks super healthy and low-calorie is not your best pick.

31 Union Square West
@16th St.
(212) 675-9500
www.bluewatergrillnyc.com

Craft

Urban Skinny Bonus
This place always has fish and always has great salads, so you can enjoy the scene and still stay skinny.

Urban Skinny Picks
Start with a Mixed Lettuce or Arugula and Lemon Salad, 2 tablespoons of dressing, for 100 calories and any one of the roasted fish entrees.

AND

Half of any one of the roasted or braised veggie sides

AND

Half of the pureed squash side
Total: 500 calories

Urban Skinny Heads-Up
Steelhead trout is an additional 100 calories.

43 E. 19th St.
@Park Ave. S. and Broadway
(212) 780-0880
www.craftrestaurant.com

Eataly

Urban Skinny Bonus

There is no shortage of variety at this mega-foodie haven. It is an experience like no other. Choose from a variety of restaurants under one roof.

Urban Skinny Picks

If you're drawn to La Pizza restaurant, go for it. Share a thin-crusted Margherita pie with a pal and split a Misticanza Salad with the dressing on the side.

OR

Try Il Pesce's filet of the day or some clams and the half shell so you can indulge in a glass of Italian vino as well. Insalata Romana with the dressing on the side has a bit of cheese so have that too for a 550-calorie meal.

Urban Skinny Heads-Up

Eataly has many food stands including chocolate, gelato, and a place to grab some cheese and meat. You can sip a glass of Prosecco while you grocery shop. Be careful not to have bites and drinks while you wander through because before you know it you'll have eaten a meal's worth of snacks before you sit down to dine.

And lines are often long for a table so stay strong and don't overeat.

200 Fifth Ave.
(646) 398-5100
www.eatalyny.com

Markt

Urban Skinny Heads-Up

Skip the bread and have a Belgian beer for a treat at 150 calories.

Urban Skinny Picks

Fresh Tomato Soup and Mussels (any of the mussel dishes except the ones made with cream), and 1 piece of bread to dip, unless you have the beer

OR

Simple Salad with Belgian Endive, 2 tablespoons of dressing, and Fruits de Mer and a Belgian beer
Both 500 calories

676 6th Ave.
@ W. 21st St. (northeast corner)
(212) 727-3314
www.marktrestaurant.com

Union Square Café

Urban Skinny Bonus
You can pick on olives instead of the bread basket, which is great if you walk in the door starving. A small olive is only 5 calories.

Urban Skinny Picks
In the winter try the Sliced Cara Cara Orange with Fennel Vinaigrette, Toasted Pine Nuts, Mint, and Ricotta Salata to start, 125 calories.

Opt for the Tuna Tartar as your entree from the appetizer list. It's a nice 4-ounce serving with a fennel cracker, 200 calories.

Have a nice glass of wine all for less than 500 calories.

OR

Go on Tuesday for the Filet Mignon of Tuna special (6-ounce portion), 250 calories. Request a side of steamed veggies. Start with a simple vegetable salad with dressing on the side for 100 calories. A glass of wine rounds you out at 500 calories.

21 E. 16th St., between 5th Ave. and Union Square
(212) 243-4020
www.unionsquarecafe.com

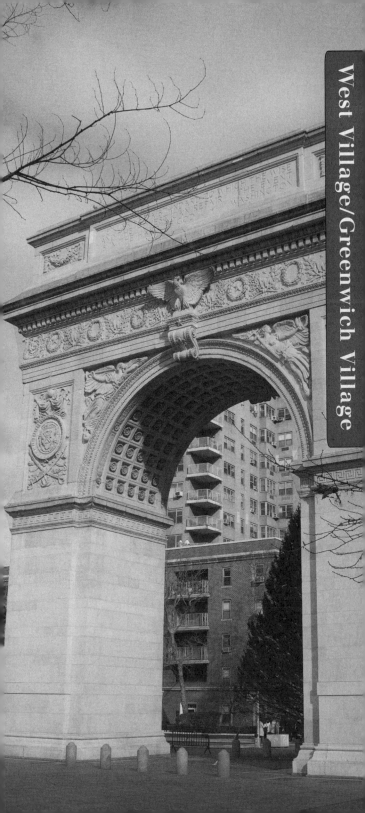

Agave

Urban Skinny Heads-Up

There are some seriously calorie-heavy appetizers, which means most are best for sharing. Choose the *side order* of the guacamole and have a taste instead of a full appetizer size. And watch out for the tequila— it's 100 calories a shot!

Urban Skinny Appetizer Pick

Tuna Tostaditas, 100–150 calories each

Urban Skinny Entree Picks

Chile Bronzed Salmon Salad with Avocado Crema on the side (instead of dressing)

3 Shrimp and Corn Tacos, 450 calories

140 7th Ave. S
(212) 989-2100
www.agaveny.com

Urban Insight: If you have 10 average-sized chips and you truly dip, not dunk, them into guacamole, you'll eat about ¼ cup of guacamole–about 250 calories altogether. If you dunk and really load your chips up, you're eating more like 550 calories–an entire meal's worth of calories for many people.

Urban Skinny Picks

Have a few small oysters to start for only 75–100 calories, and make the Smoked Oil Poached Salmon your main course, for an additional 450 calories.

OR

Baby Arugula Salad, with the dressing on the side, Oven Roasted Whole Dourade, and a small piece of warm bread for under 600 calories

Urban Skinny Heads-Up

August doesn't take reservations. Make sure you don't go there starving, so that by the time you sit down you shovel in 1,500 calories fast.

The Skinny

There are appetizers on this menu—you can only have a sliver—the most popular being the Alsatian Onion Tart. It is more than 500 calories, so it's either your dinner, or you have a quarter of it to start and then just get a white fish as your main.

359 Bleecker St.
@ Charles and W. l0th
(212) 929-8727
www.augustny.com

BLT Burger

Urban Skinny Picks

Yes, a burger is an okay pick because here it's only 5 ounces precooked! Grilled Certified Black Angus Beef is a blend of brisket, chuck, short rib, and beef, which is fattier than ground sirloin. The small portion size makes it an Urban Skinny Burger Pick for 500 calories.

Classic, or The Streaker with No Bun, or the Grilled CAB Burger, lettuce, tomato, onion, bell pepper, avocado, 500 calories

470 6th Ave., between 11th and 12th Sts.
(212) 243-8226
www.bltburger.com

Urban Myth: Fat makes you fat.

Urban Skinny: Fat, fortunately, is great. It actually helps you lose weight because it makes meals more satisfying and keeps you full longer. Include a little fat in every meal. A tablespoon of olive oil or a tablespoon of peanut butter is only about 100 calories. Why eat dry toast or salad with just vinegar if you don't have to?

Corner Bistro

Urban Skinny Picks

Grilled Chicken Sandwich, small handful of fries, 550 calories

Burger with a bun (no fries), 8 ounces uncooked, so 6 ounces cooked, 600 calories

A bowl of chili is 400 calories and a great source of fiber.

Urban Skinny Heads-Up

Do not order the Bistro burger—that has bacon and cheese, which would mean almost 300 extra calories, on top of the 600!

The Skinny

Some say this is the best burger in the city and while it's not the "healthiest" menu in town, from a calorie standpoint, you can pull it off.

331 W. 4th St. @ Jane St.
(212) 242-9502
www.cornerbistrony.com

Da Silvano

Urban Skinny Bonus

You can order mussels by portion size and pasta as half orders, so it's easy to eat small here.

Urban Skinny Picks

Start with a fresh mixed salad with 2 tablespoons of dressing, for 100 calories. Add the Grilled Prawns with Veggies for 350 calories, and 1 small piece of bread for 50–100 calories and your meal is 500–550 calories.

OR

Combine 2 appetizers. The Bread Salad with 2 table-spoons dressing on the side is 200 calories. Ask for ¼ pound of Steamed Mussels for 150 calories, and one glass of wine for another 150 calories, and you have a 500–calorie meal.

OR

Start with a Fresh Mixed Salad with 2 tablespoons of dressing for 100 calories. Get a half order of Whole Wheat Penne Pasta with Pesto, which is 350 calories, and you have a total meal for 450 calories.

260 6th Ave., between Houston & Bleecker Sts.
(212) 982-2343
www.dasilvano.com

Dell'anima

Urban Skinny Bonus
This is a great place for bits and bites and a full meal. The pasta portions are perfect Urban Skinny size. You can sit at the bar and have a light bite and a glass of wine.

Urban Skinny Pick
Arugula Salad with Shaved Reggiano Cheese and Lemon, with dressing on the side, 100–150 calories

Pick a pasta portion without cream sauce options, and you get away with 500 calories for a bowl.

Urban Skinny Treat
Bruschetta here has several toppings options. Each piece of bruschetta with a topping is no more than 50 calories, so you can have a glass of wine, a salad, and 5 bruschetta pieces for less than 600 calories.

38 8th Ave.
(212) 366-6633
www.dellanima.com

Employees Only

Urban Skinny Appetizer Picks

Mixed Green Salad (under the Sides Section), with dressing on the side (2 tablespoons is 100 calories)

OR

Cucumber and Radish Salad, 50 calories
Be sure to get the Vinaigrette and Caraway Cracker Dressing on the side, and use 1 tablespoon for 100 calories.

Urban Skinny Picks

Elk Loin, 6 ounces precooked, 4½ ounces cooked, 250 calories

Broccoli Rabe, 350 calories

OR

Organic Chicken—take off the skin, stick with white meat, and skip the dark meat. Four ounces is 200 calories. It's served with Brussel Sprouts and Potato, for a total of 400–450 calories.

OR

3 to 4 oysters appetizer, 100 calories

Whole roasted Rainbow Trout, 7 ounces—omit the skin, served with Frisée salad, for 300 calories and one glass of wine OR one piece of the Kajmak Cheese Bread from the bread basket for a total of 550 calories.

Urban Skinny Pitfall

The Polenta Fritter and Foie Gras Mousse

Urban Skinny Tip
Skip the starch and grab a glass of wine and enjoy the fireplace.

Urban Skinny Extra
Entertain yourself with the psychic, not dessert, after dinner, for a real treat.

510 Hudson St.
(212) 242-3021
www.employeesonlynyc.com

Urban Insight: If you plan to drink, you don't get to eat as much. We know you're going to hit the town every once in a while. But remember that the more you drink, the less you should eat. (We do not, however, encourage you to drink heavily—especially on an empty stomach!) You might even find that since you only have so many calories to spend, you wind up forgoing the booze for food.

Gotham Bar and Grill

Urban Skinny Bonus
Great for lunch!

Urban Skinny Starter
Start with the Baby Organic Mixed Green Salad, aged sherry and extra-virgin olive oil dressing on the side, and use 2 tablespoons for 100 calories.

Urban Skinny Entree Picks
Roasted Scottish Salmon, Braised Fennel, Tomato Confit, Spinach, and Lemon Oil with Warm Fennel Vinaigrette

OR

New Zealand Pink Snapper, Artichoke Hearts, Haricots Verts and Braised Shallots, with Green and Black Cerignola Olive Sauce
All 500 calories

12 E. 12th St., between 5th Ave. and University Place
(212) 620-4020
www.gothambarandgrill.com

Havana Alma De Cuba

Urban Skinny Heads-Up
The portions of fish are large, so order half portions.

Urban Skinny Sides
Habana Salad with either Avocado or dressing on the side,100 calories

A small Black Bean Soup,150–200 calories

Urban Skinny Entree Picks
Half order of Ropa Vieja, 400–450 calories

OR

Half order of the Red Snapper, a 10-ounce portion, so cut to 5 ounces, served with Avocado and Sofrito Sauce, 250 calories

OR

Half order of Salmon Santa Clara, sauce on the side, served with Rice and Shrimp, 375 calories

Mix and match for a 500-calorie dinner.

Urban Skinny Extra
A glass of signature sangria is 150 calories, so skip the starch here and enjoy.

94 Christopher St., between Bleecker and Bedford Sts.
(212) 242-3800
www.havananyc.com

Urban Skinny Bonus

Like many places, you can substitute egg whites for eggs, which saves you calories and can accommodate gluten-intolerant diners.

Urban Skinny Picks

Mushroom Omelet with Baby Portobello, Tomato, Fontina, and Herbs, served with mixed greens for under 350–400 calories

OR

Eggs Florentine (if you order hollandaise on the side), 350 calories plus 75 calories per tablespoon of sauce

Urban Skinny Add-Ons

150 calories will get you a Bloody Mary or use 100 calories for a slice of wheat toast.

100 W. Houston St., between LaGuardia Place and Thompson St.
(212) 254-7000
www.ctrnyc.com

John's Pizzeria

Urban Skinny Bonus
They offer a whole-wheat crust and plenty of veggie toppings!

Urban Skinny Picks
Start with a house salad to add volume to your meal.

AND

Have a Whole Wheat Margherita Pizza at 200 calories per slice. Add a little grilled chicken to boost your protein intake, for an additional 35 extra calories per slice.

278 Bleecker St., between Jones and Morton
(212) 243-1680
www.johnspizzerianyc.com

Urban Myth: Sugar turns to fat. "Carbohydrate" is just a longer word for sugar.

Urban Skinny: People think bagels, pasta, and potatoes turn to fat. Everyone is on an anti-carb kick because they buy into this misconception. The bottom line is, anything eaten in excess adds extra pounds onto your body. There's no discriminating: The only thing that causes weight gain is extra calories. Carbs—which are sugar, it's true—don't add to your weight-loss challenge any more than any other nutrient does.

Lupa

Urban Skinny Bonus
You can have pasta! If you have pasta, you shouldn't also have wine. But Lupa serves a carafe of wine that gives two people a nice 4-ounce taste and is just 100 calories, so in this one instance, have a small glass.

Urban Skinny Picks
Try the Linguini with Razor Clams or the Spaghetti with Pomodoro, for a simple but delicious dish at 400 calories.

OR

Bucatini alla Amatriciana or the Ricotta Gnocchi with Sausage & Fennel, 500 calories

If you like, start with a simple vegetable salad. Add on for dressing, 100 calories for 2 tablespoons.

Urban Skinny Tip
Skip the bread basket. It shouldn't be too hard, since it is not warm.

170 Thompson St.
between Houston and Bleecker Sts.
(212) 982-5089
www.luparestaurant.com

Mas Farmhouse

Urban Skinny Bonus
Most chicken and fish entrees are 3–6 ounces, so portions are appropriate on all entrees. Stick with the choices that are mostly grilled or roasted and that have minimal sauces. Most will be less than 400 calories.

Urban Skinny Heads-Up
The menu changes daily so we can't make specific recommendations. There is no bread basket so it's easy to say "no thank you" when the waiter asks if you would like a piece of bread.

Urban Skinny Picks
Order a grilled entree and add a side of sautéed veggies for a 500–550-calorie dinner.

Urban Skinny Tip
They offer a complimentary glass of champagne upon arrival, which has just 75 calories a flute. Enjoy it and skip the 150-calorie glass of wine.

39 Downing St.
between Bedford and Varick Sts.
(212) 255-1790
www.masfarmhouse.com

Otto

Urban Skinny Bonus

It's a great place for sharing, so you can taste a lot of little things, especially if you pick antipasto starters. Pizzas are small so you can have a slice with a salad and you'll still be Urban Skinny.

Urban Skinny Picks

Arugula or romaine salad as a filler at the beginning of your meal is a must; otherwise, you'll end up eating 4 slices of pizza.

Otto slice with veggies, 200 calories

If you are going for antipasto as a meal, stick with mostly the vegetables and fish and garnish with 1 selection of cheese. Fish picks will be about 150 calories, veggies 100 calories, and your cheese is 150 calories.

Urban Skinny Pitfall

Use your judgment on the oil in some of these antipasto choices. Oil means calories.

1 5th Ave.
(212) 995-9559
www.ottopizzeria.com

The Standard Grill

Urban Skinny Bonus
The raw bar options make this fun for sharing.

Urban Skinny Picks
Opt for the Bibb salad with the dressing on the side and choose fish from the grill section as your main course.

Urban Skinny Pitfall
Avoid the fondue if possible and watch out for cured meats. They can be a big draw, but can add up very quickly. One ounce of sopressata or chorizo is 75 to 100 calories.

848 Washington St. @ 13th St.
(212) 645-4100
www.thestandardgrill.com

Sushi Samba

Urban Skinny Picks
Field Green Salad and the Yellowtail Sashimi Ceviche, 125 calories

AND

Rockfish a la Plancha, delicious and light, 300 calories

Urban Skinny Heads-Up
Some of the most popular rolls (Samba 7 and El Topo) are a little richer than your typical roll and are served in 7–8 pieces instead of the traditional 6 pieces. Count 60–70 calories per piece in this case.

87 7th Ave. S
@ corner of Barrow St.
(212) 691-7885
www.sushisamba.com

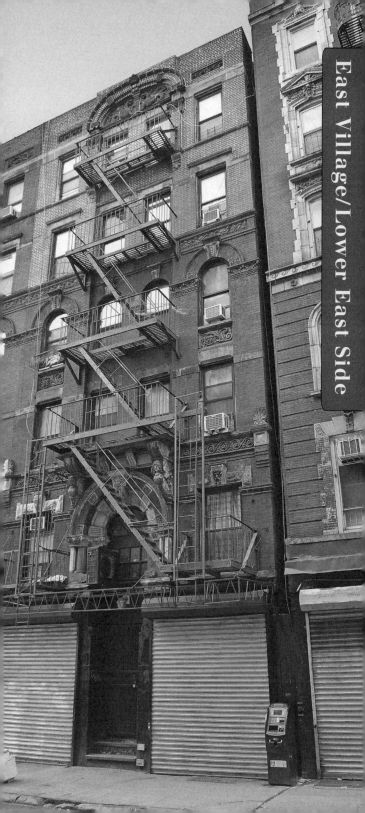

Apizz

Urban Skinny Picks

Insalata Verde (without dressing), Whole Roasted
Fish, and a glass of wine, 500 calories

OR

A salad with dressing on the side, share a Mushroom
Polenta and Whole Roasted Fish, 500 calories

**217 Eldridge St., between Stanton and
Rivington Sts.**
(212) 253-9199
www.apizz.com

Urban Myth: Weigh yourself every day.

Urban Skinny: Salt, hormones, getting off
a plane, and, uh, how shall we say this, not
taking a poop can make it look like you're
failing, but you're not. Weigh yourself once a
week at the same time, and assess your overall
progress monthly so you don't get discouraged.
Take measurements and know how your
clothing fits. And check your body composition,
because a pound of fat takes up more space
than a pound of muscle.

Back Forty (Brunch)

Urban Skinny Picks

Poached Eggs and Baby Green Wheat, served with toast, 450 calories
> Order toast without butter!

OR

Grass-Fed Burger on a bun, 500–550 calories

Add the Butterhead Lettuce Salad with Fried Shallots for 150 calories with 2 tablespoons of dressing.

For a brunch total of 600–650 calories; brunch is two meals combined, not one.

Urban Skinny Tip

The burger is not served with fries. They charge $2 extra for the fries, which makes it easy to skip them.

190 Ave. B @ E. 12th St.
(212) 388-1990
www.backfortynyc.com

Barrio Chino

Three Small Tacos make this place a great choice for Mexican.

Chicken or Fish Tacos, 75 calories each, 225 total

AND

Ensalada de Nopales, no dressing, but keep avocado and fresh cheese, 250 calories

OR

Ceviche and Ensalada de Calamari, no dressing, 300 calories

One grapefruit margarita, 200 calories

OR

Cazuela De Mariscos Seafood Stew with calamari and shrimp, served with bread

253 Broome St., between Orchard and Ludlow Sts.
(212) 228-6710
www.barriochinonyc.com

Beauty & Essex

Urban Skinny Bonus
Great for sharing

Urban Skinny Picks
Have a typical raw bar experience here, and be sure to try the tomato tartar for just 150 calories. Pick at some crudo, sashimi, and shrimp with friends for another 150 calories. The lobster taco is small, but fried so you can make that your main at just 150 calories and share some grilled asparagus with the crowd.

OR

If you aren't in a sharing mood try the tuna entree, which is the best choice at 350 calories.

146 Essex St.
(212) 614-0146
www.beautyandessex.com

DBGB

Urban Skinny Picks

Chop-Chop Salad, appetizer size, 50 calories before dressing; use 2 tablespoons of dressing for 150 calories.

Small order of Red Curry Mussels, 300 calories

OR

Large Chop-Chop Salad with Lobster, 400 calories Four ounces of lobster is 250 calories before dressing. Use 3 tablespoons of dressing for the salad since it is an entree.

One piece of bread from the bread basket is 100 calories.

OR

Yankee Burger, 6 ounces precooked and 4½ ounces cooked, open-faced on just half the bun, 400 calories

Skip the fries and substitute for the Ratatouille, 100 calories.

Urban Skinny Heads-Up

They are famous for their sausage, but it is very high in calories. If you must have a taste, do just that but avoid it as an entree.

299 Bowery St., between Houston and 1st Sts.
(212) 933-5300
www.danielnyc.com

Stanton Social

Urban Skinny Bonus

There is no bread basket, and small servings allow you to sample a bunch of things, so it's great to go with a group of people.

Urban Skinny Picks

The famous French Onion Soup Dumplings, 75 calories each

Red Snapper Tacos, 75 calories each

Tuna Nori Roll, 50 calories each

Pierogies, 75 calories each

The Kobe Slider is a great way to get your taste for a burger satisfied in a controlled portion, for 200 calories.

Add a few dishes from the raw bar for a scant amount of calories:
    Little Neck Clams, 10 calories each
    Shrimp, 25 calories each

Urban Skinny Pitfall

It's easy to lose track of how much you are eating, so pay attention!

99 Stanton St.
between Ludlow and Orchard Sts.
(212) 995-0099
www.thestantonsocial.com

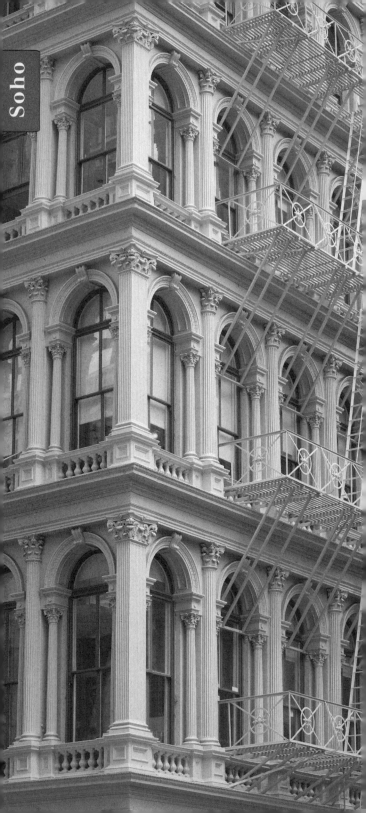

Aquagrill

Urban Skinny Bonus

The bread basket isn't dropped on the table, but offered up one piece at a time, making it easy to say no.

Urban Skinny Picks

A Green Salad with dressing on the side

OR

Some raw bar oysters—the large ones are 40 calories each, the small ones are 10 calories each.

AND

Grilled, poached, or roasted white fish with steamed veggies on the side

AND

A glass of wine

All in, just 500 calories, or if you pick the salmon, it's 600 calories.

210 Spring St.
@ 6th Ave.
(212) 274-0505
www.aquagrill.com

Balthazar

Urban Skinny Brunch Picks

Eggs Benedict, Florentine, or Norwegian, with the hollandaise sauce on the side; with no sauce, 370 calories; 1 tablespoon of sauce costs you 75 calories.

Small Fruit Salad, 100 calories

Urban Skinny Dinner Pick

Salad Niçoise, dressing on the side, 400 calories

80 Spring St., between Broadway and Crosby
(212) 965-1414
www.balthazarny.com

Urban Insight: A busy workday and stress can sometimes distract you during the day and make you forget to, or choose not to, eat. Once you wind down, you'll blow the diet because hunger will take control of your willpower. If it doesn't get you that night, you'll chow big time the following morning.

Boqueria

Urban Skinny Bonus

The menu here changes, but the nice thing is that it's all small plates, so you can get a group of people together and just share a bunch of things to get to a perfect 500- or 600-calorie meal.

Urban Skinny Dinner Picks

Gambas al Ajillo (Ruby Red Shrimp), 150–200 calories each

Stuffed Dates, 50 calories each

Baby Squid, 150 calories each

Pimientos de Padron (little green peppers), 100 calories

Seared Lamb, 200–250 calories

Quesos (cheese), 1-inch cube, 100 calories

Paella is served for two, so 1 cup (one fist) is 250 calories.

Glass of Sangria, 150 calories

Keep a tally of what you're eating—taking one taste of each thing until you hit the 500-calorie mark. Order slowly!

171 Spring St.
@ W. Broadway
(212) 343-4255
(Also in Flatiron @ 53 W. 19th St., between 5th and 6th Aves.; 212-255-4160)
www.boquerianyc.com

Dos Caminos

Urban Skinny Picks

Ceviche to start, just under 150 calories

AND

Mahimahi Fish Tacos with corn *not* flour tortillas, 400 calories

OR

Pescado Veracruzano, 300 calories

One order of Guacamole is 800 calories. If there are four of you, and you ask for crudite instead of chips, skip the ceviche and have a quarter of the order.

Urban Skinny Pitfalls

You have to avoid the chips, and a margarita on the rocks is 200 calories.

475 W. Broadway, between Houston and Prince Sts.
(212) 277-4300
www.doscaminos.com

Ed's Lobster Bar

Urban Skinny Bonus

This place has great pickles, and while they're high in sodium, they have only a few calories.

Urban Skinny Appetizer Picks

Raw Bar or Shrimp Cocktail, about 50 calories a piece

Urban Skinny Entree Picks

A Lobster Roll could be 600 or 700 calories, so skip the fries, cut the roll in half and share it or save it, and have a Bibb Salad with 2 tablespoons of dressing. If half won't do, make this meal brunch—combining your breakfast calories and lunch calories—and eat the whole thing.

OR

Just have a 1½-pound Whole Steamed Lobster for 250–300 calories (no butter, just squeeze lemon).

222 Lafayette St., between Kenmare and Spring
(212) 343-3236
www.lobsterbarnyc.com

Lure

Urban Skinny Bonus
They have lots of seafood, raw and sushi picks, and will steam your veggies upon request.

Urban Skinny Appetizer Picks
All 100 calories

Ceviche or Carpaccio (2.5–3 ounces)

Lure House Salad

3 large oysters or 5 small oysters

Urban Skinny Note
We did not list the Crispy Blue Point Oysters, which are fried and sauced to calorie torture.

Opt for one of the steamed fish entrees (6-ounce portion) for 200–250 calories. Some dishes are served with a starch, so add an additional 100 calories if you partake.

Urban Skinny Pitfall
The bread basket is filled with fresh, hot mini-pullman loaves, 200 calories each.

142 Mercer St. (downstairs)
@ Prince St.
(212) 431-7676
www.lurefishbar.com

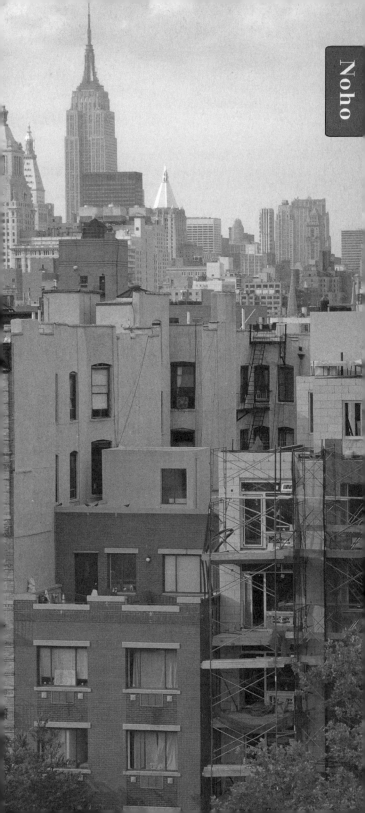

Noho Star

Urban Skinny Bonus
It's great for breakfast because it has heart-healthy foods, such as almonds and ground flax seeds.

Urban Skinny Picks
Soft Boiled Eggs with Asparagus and Dry Toast, 400 calories

OR

Greek Yogurt with Honey and Toasted Almonds or Ground Flax Seeds, 300 calories

Request honey on the side and drizzle on 1 tablespoon.

OR

Steel-cut Oatmeal with Raisins and Hazelnuts, 450 calories

330 Lafayette St.
(212) 925-0070
www.nohostar.com

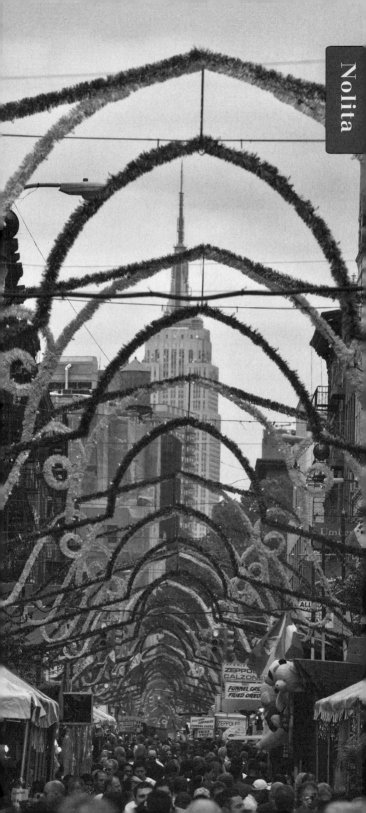

Public (Brunch)

Urban Skinny Heads-Up
Brunch means you're combining your lunch and breakfast into one meal, for 600–700 calories, which is okay on a weekend.

Urban Skinny Bonus
Brunch is an occasion to break a rule. It's is a bigger meal so no need to substitute your bread for a cocktail—you can enjoy both.

Urban Skinny Picks
2 Poached Eggs on Sourdough Toast with Tomatoes and Mushrooms, 450 calories

OR

Tea-smoked Salmon, Spinach, and Poached Eggs on Toasted Sourdough with Yuzu Hollandaise, 550 calories

Add 70 calories per tablespoon of hollandaise.

For just breakfast: Granola and yogurt parfait, 350–450 calories

Urban Skinny Tip
Be sure to get hollandaise on the side and dip your fork.

Urban Skinny 100-Calorie Add-On
Mimosa

210 Elizabeth St.
between Prince and Spring Sts.
(212) 343-7011
www.public-nyc.com

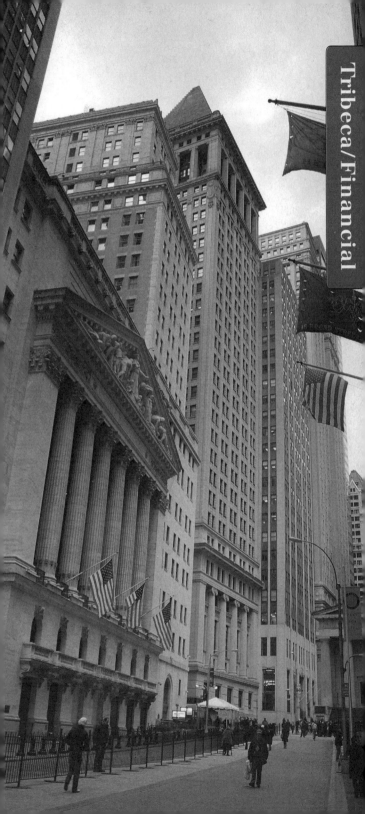

Bouley Restaurant

Urban Skinny Bonus

There are lots of good fish picks at this trendy hotspot.

Urban Skinny Picks

Choose the Bibb salad to start. If you want a glass of wine consider one of the seafood appetizers as your main or try Black Sea Bass Entree with spinach and buckwheat and skip the vino.

163 Duane Street @ Hudson St.
(212) 964-2525
www.davidbouley.com

Urban Myth: Everyone turns to food to deal with stress.

Urban Skinny: More often it's chronic dieters who eat to de-stress, while non-dieters might turn to the gym. Dieters spend a lot of time depriving themselves of their favorite foods, so when they hit a wall they say "screw it" and shove five cookies in with absolutely no thought. When living an Urban Skinny lifestyle you won't be depriving yourself of anything, so you'll be less likely to turn to food for comfort in rough times.

Dylan Prime

Urban Skinny Pick

Go for the 7-ounce filet mignon for 350 calories and a side of asparagus for 150 calories, or a glass of cabernet for 150 calories.

Urban Skinny Heads-Up

Good steak doesn't need any sauces or chapeaux. Sauces are often hundreds of calories.

62 Laight St.
(212) 334-4783
www.dylanprime.com

Urban Insight: At a steak house, they usually tell you up front on the menu how big a piece of meat you're ordering. Remember that this number includes the bone and fat, before the meat is cooked. Once it's cooked, protein shrinks 25 percent. Eight ounces on the menu will be six ounces on the plate.

Hale and Hearty

Urban Skinny Bonus

Choice, choice, choice. If this is your lunch go-to, you can mix it up every day. There are great soup and sandwich combos (half sandwich and an 8-ounce soup) and lots of salad picks.

Urban Skinny Heads-Up

If you go for a lighter-calorie sandwich, you can opt for a higher-calorie soup. Soups are labeled for vegetarians and dairy free.

Some 80–90 calories per 8-ounce cup:

10-Vegetable

Gazpacho

Ginger Carrot

Tomato Vegetable

Ginger Carrot Artichoke

Tomato Eggplant

Tomato Florentine

Half sandwiches:

Turkey on 7-grain roll, 200 calories plus 100 calories per packet of mayo

Ham and Cheddar, 250 calories

Turkey and Cranberry with Aioli, 250 calories

Roast Beef and Mozzarella, 300 calories

55 Broad St.
@ Beaver St.
(212) 509-4100
www.haleandhearty.com

Landmarc

Urban Skinny Bonus
All sandwiches are served with field greens, but be sure to request dressing on the side.

Urban Skinny Picks
Any "gourmet" sandwich, have half, 350–400 calories Add the side salad with 2 tablespoons of dressing for 500 calories total.

OR

Small order of Mussels with White Wine or Provencal Sauce (20–30 mussels) and a piece of bread from the bread basket. Add on either the field greens or chopped salad with 2 tablespoons vinaigrette for 400 calories, which is good for lunch.

OR

Tuna Niçoise Salad with Potato, Egg, and Anchovy and 3 tablespoons of dressing, 500 calories

179 W. Broadway, between Leonard and Worth Sts.
(212) 343-3883
(Also @ the Time Warner Center, 10 Columbus Circle, 3rd floor; (212) 823-6123
www.landmarc-restaurant.com

Nobu

Urban Skinny Bonus
You can get a bunch of appetizers and try a lot of different things and share or order your own specialties.

Urban Skinny Picks
Sashimi Tacos (3 tacos), 75 calories each, 225 calories per order

Kushiyaki (2 skewers):
Chicken, 150 calories

Beef, 200 calories

Salmon, 200 calories

Shrimp, 120 calories

Rolls: 40–60 calories per piece

OR

Start with a salad and have the Black Cod with Miso, 350 calories.

105 Hudson St.
@ Franklin St.
(212) 219-0500
www.noburestaurants.com

Vino Vino

Urban Skinny Bonus

Small plates are the way to go here, so even if you're not sharing, you can get lots of little nibbles to make a meal.

Urban Skinny Picks

This is a wine bar, so enjoy a glass of wine for 150 calories.

Trentino/Bresaola, Parmigiano Reggiano, and Baby Arugula, finished with White Truffle Oil and the Shaved Brussel Sprouts Salad, with Pecorino and Walnuts, finished with extra-virgin olive oil and lemon

211 W. Broadway
(212) 925-8510
www.vinovino.net

Butter Cup

One cupcake, 350–400 calories
www.buttercupbakeshop.com

Crumbs

Big cupcakes, 800 calories
Normal size, 400 calories
Minis, 125 calories
www.crumbs.com

Magnolia Bakery

One cupcake, 350–400 calories
One homemade cookie, 125 calories
www.magnoliacupcakes.com

Make My Cake

One cupcake, 500 calories
One Red Velvet cupcake, 600 calories
www.makemycake.us

Pinkberry

Urban Skinny Bonus
They weigh each cup so you can count on your serving and calories being accurate.

Small: 5 ounces, 125 calories

Medium: 8 ounces, 200 calories

Large: 12 ounces, 325 calories

Fruit toppings: 10–20 calories each

Fruit is fresh, not frozen or canned.

www.pinkberry.com

Red Mango

Urban Skinny Bonus
This treat gives you 10 percent of your daily requirement of calcium. It also contains live and active probiotic cultures and is certified by the National Yogurt Association. It's made with kosher ingredients.

Small: 4 ounces, 100 calories

Regular: 8 ounces, 200 calories

Large: 12 ounces, 300 calories

www.redmangousa.com

Tasti D-Lite

Urban Skinny Heads-Up

Most flavors are 20 calories per ounce, but peanut butter is 25 calories per ounce.

In a cup:

Small: 4 ounces, 80 calories

Medium/regular: 8 ounces, 160 calories

Large: 12 ounces, 240 calories

Pint: 16 ounces, 320 calories

Make your topping sprinkles since there is no fruit to choose, and add 50 calories to your cup.

Urban Skinny Pitfall

These guys don't weigh each cup so the portions may not be exact and the calories may be higher or lower than listed. You might think you're doing well with a small, but if you add in a cone and toppings, you're at 300 calories before you know it.

Urban Skinny Tips

Order a small, so if calorie count is off you won't kill a day.

Cake cones have fewer calories than a sugar cones: 15 calories versus 60 calories.

www.tastidlite.com

Vinaigrette, 2 tablespoons

Small bowl of fruit or glass of orange juice

One cup sautéed veggies

Small dinner roll

Piece of bread (dip your bread in oil, add another 100 calories)

½ cup rice, pasta, or potato

10 small tortilla chips

¼ cup guacamole

½ bowl edamame

10 large olives

Cheese added to a salad

Glass of champagne

Glass of Port

Latte

2 strips bacon

¼ cup hummus

½ pita

2 pieces sushi

3-ounce lobster tail

A New York Slice at most places with cheese, sauce, and veggies, 500 calories

New York bagel with cream cheese, 600 calories

Dirty Water Dog (hot dog from a cart), 200 calories

Pretzel from a cart, 600 calories

A bag of roasted nuts from a cart, 400 calories

Danielle Schupp, RD, counsels more than fifty clients a week from her office at one of New York's top fitness clubs, the Reebok Sports Club/NY. She has appeared on *Entertainment Tonight* and refereed an employee weight-loss challenge on *Live with Regis and Kelly*. Her weight management advice has been featured in *Self*, *Marie Claire*, *Redbook,* and *Forbes*.

Stephanie Krikorian is a celebrity ghostwriter and pop-culture blogger. Her first career was in the TV news business. She has covered two Olympic Games, the Grammy Awards' Red Carpet, and dozens of international and domestic news stories. She is a travel buff who has been to six continents.

About the Authors